Yaneir Wilson Laurencio
Nadiezha Valton Masso
Lesbia Marino Madariaga

LUNG CARCINOMA

Yaneir Wilson Laurencio
Nadiezha Valton Masso
Lesbia Marino Madariaga

LUNG CARCINOMA

A CLINICOPATHOLOGIC CHARACTERIZATION IN NECROTIC DECEDENTS

ScienciaScripts

Imprint
Any brand names and product names mentioned in this book are subject to trademark, brand or patent protection and are trademarks or registered trademarks of their respective holders. The use of brand names, product names, common names, trade names, product descriptions etc. even without a particular marking in this work is in no way to be construed to mean that such names may be regarded as unrestricted in respect of trademark and brand protection legislation and could thus be used by anyone.

Cover image: www.ingimage.com

This book is a translation from the original published under ISBN 978-620-0-01355-2.

Publisher:
Sciencia Scripts
is a trademark of
Dodo Books Indian Ocean Ltd. and OmniScriptum S.R.L publishing group

120 High Road, East Finchley, London, N2 9ED, United Kingdom
Str. Armeneasca 28/1, office 1, Chisinau MD-2012, Republic of Moldova, Europe
Managing Directors: Ieva Konstantinova, Victoria Ursu
info@omniscriptum.com

Printed at: see last page
ISBN: 978-620-8-61021-0

ACKNOWLEDGMENTS

To my family, the most important thing in my life.

To my mother, for her understanding and help in difficult moments; she has taught me to see the sun when the sky was gray. Thank you for instilling in me everything I am, for the values and principles that have made me try to be a better person and professional.

To my children for being a source of inspiration and for their love present in every moment of my life. To them, for their patience and unconditional support. Thank you.

SUMMARY

Lung cancer is a chronic non-communicable disease and is currently the leading cause of cancer-related death in the Americas. The highest incidence and mortality rates for this disease occur in North America and Cuba, while the lowest rates are recorded in the Caribbean. The aim of this study was to characterize the necrotized deceased with the clinicopathological diagnosis of lung carcinoma in the General Teaching Hospital "Dr. Agostinho Neto" of Guantánamo. For this purpose, a descriptive cross-sectional, retrospective study was conducted on 114 deceased with the clinicopathological diagnosis of lung carcinoma in the period given between 2017-2020. In the study conducted, the most affected age group was 51-70 years old with 55.3%, most were from urban origin with 84.2%, non-smokers with 93% and with no family history of lung carcinoma with 91.2%. The greatest number of deceased were workers and retirees with 67.51% and 24.6%, respectively. The most frequent histologic type was squamous cell carcinoma with 45.6%. In the distribution by clinical stage, stage III disease was most frequent with 87.7%. The necrotized deceased with lung carcinoma at the General Teaching Hospital "Dr. Agostinho Neto" in the period under study were characterized, taking into account sociodemographic factors, the most frequent histological type and its relationship with the clinical stage at the time of diagnosis.

CONTENTS

INTRODUCTION

The structure of the lungs is ingeniously formed so that it can fulfill its primary function, the exchange of gases between the inspired air and the blood. The right lung is divided into three lobes and the left lung into only two, the equivalent of the middle lobe is the lingula.

The airways (right and left main bronchi) start from the trachea and then branch by successive dichotomies, giving rise to smaller and smaller airways. [(1)]

The respiratory system originates as a ventral medial diverticulum of the pharyngeal wall (foregut), immediately caudal to the hypo bronchial eminence, termed the respiratory diverticulum or pulmonary sketch, in the middle of the fourth week (25 somites). Thus, the inner lining epithelium of the larynx, trachea and bronchi, like that of the lungs, is of endodermal (parenchymal) origin. The cartilaginous, muscular and connective tissue components of the trachea and lungs, on the other hand, are derived from the asplastic mesoderm (stroma). [(2)]

The two main components of the lung parenchyma are the bronchi, bronchioles (airways) and alveoli. The alveoli are lined by type 1 and type 2 (granular) pneumocytes; the latter produce surfactant and are the main proliferative component after alveolar injury. [(2)]

The alveolar walls contain capillaries whose basement membrane fuses with that of the alveolar epithelium to form a single alveolar capillary membrane. The main cells of the epithelium of the bronchi and bronchioles are basal cells, neuroendocrine cells (Kulchitsky type), hair cells, serous cells, Clara cells, and goblet cells. [(1,2)]

Goblet and hair cells decrease in number as the terminal bronchioles are approached, while the number of Clara cells increases proportionally. Clara cells have a secretory function and represent the main progenitor cells after bronchiolar injury. [1,2]

The microscopic structure of the alveolar walls (or alveolar septa) is formed, from the blood to the air, by the following components: Capillary endothelium and basement membrane, the alveolar interstitium, consisting of fine elastic fibers, small collagen bundles, few fibroblast-like cells, smooth muscle cells, mast cells, and infrequent mononuclear cells, is most conspicuous in the thicker portions of the alveolar septum.[3]

The alveolar walls are not solid, but are perforated by numerous Kohn's pores, which allow the passage of air, bacteria and exudates between adjacent alveoli. Alveolar macrophages, which are usually free within the alveolar space. [3]

Cancer is a group of diseases characterized by the uncontrolled proliferation of genetically damaged cells. These cells have two fundamental characteristics that make them potentially dangerous for the organism. Firstly, they reproduce without responding to regulation and control mechanisms and, secondly, they invade regions or areas that correspond to other cells. [4]

Cancer is caused by somatically acquired genetic changes, sometimes associated with the existence of hereditary predispositions. It is a genetic disease that occurs at the cellular level, as a result of the accumulation of mutations in genes that control the division and death of cells [5].

These genetic alterations are the main initiating factor and are also responsible for tumor progression. Cancers are classified according to the tissue and cell type from which they originate.

Those originating from epithelial cells are called carcinomas. The vast majority of cancers belong to this group (about 90%), which includes those that affect many of the internal organs, including the lung. (5)

At the turn of the 20th century, lung carcinoma was a medical curiosity. Lung carcinoma at the beginning of the present century caused 1% of all deaths, but this has progressively increased and today it is one of the leading causes of death from cancer in the world. Its relative frequency has also increased with respect to other neoplasms (6).

Lung carcinoma is currently the third most frequent type of cancer and the leading cause of cancer-related death in the Americas, with more than 324,000 new cases and nearly 262,000 deaths each year. The highest incidence and mortality rates for this disease in women are in North America and Cuba, while the lowest rates are in the Caribbean.(6)

In the lung, most of the tumors that arise are bronchogenic carcinomas (90 to 95%). Approximately 5 % are bronchial carcinoids and 2 to 5 % are mesenchymal and miscellaneous tumors. The term bronchogenic indicates that the origin of these tumors is the bronchial epithelium and sometimes the bronchiolar epithelium. (4)

If the tumor cells remain clustered in a localized isolated solid mass, it is a benign tumor. If the cells can escape from the tumor, invade adjacent tissues, pass into the bloodstream, invade lymph nodes and form secondary tumors in other distant areas, it is a malignant tumor or cancer, properly speaking. This process of dissemination of a tumor to other regions is called metastasis. [4]

The incidence of lung carcinoma, according to the 2019 report, in Spain, is estimated at 277,234 for this year, 2 % more than in 2015, when the figures for new cases were 247,000. In addition, survival in Spain continues to rise in recent times, being 53 % at 5 years, similar to that of surrounding countries.[7]

If no action is taken, it is predicted that by 2030, the number of people diagnosed with lung carcinoma will increase by 32% and rise to more than 5 million people per year in the Americas, due to an aging population, changing lifestyles and exposure to risk factors. [7]

It is valid to point out that in Cuba lung carcinoma is the first cause of death in women, but not in men, which is the second, only preceded by prostate cancer, according to the current statistical yearbook [7].

In recent years, biological knowledge of various oncological diseases has increased, largely thanks to technological developments that have enabled successful research in the molecular genetic field. [8]

This knowledge has been transferred to the clinic, in such a way that a close correlation has been established between the molecular biology of malignant neoplasms and their clinical behavior, and even more so, with the possibility of personalized therapies. [6]

The development of cancer involves the presence of several genetic alterations in cells; only one alteration is not sufficient to cause cancer. These mutations accumulate in somatic cells throughout life, so that the probability of developing cancer, in most cases, increases considerably with age. [6]

For the diagnosis of lung carcinoma there are multiple procedures, between invasive and non-invasive, which are used depending on the size and location of the tumor, the most commonly used are bronchoscopy with or without associated histological techniques (brushing, bronchial aspirate (bronchial biopsy), Computed Axial Tomography, fine needle aspiration biopsy and sputum cytology study.[9]

Foundation

Lung carcinoma is a global health problem, with an estimated annual death toll of 1.69 million according to the World Health Organization (WHO), making it the cancer with the highest number of deaths in the world. Therefore, it is considered today as one of the leading causes of death worldwide. [7]

For its part, Cuba, in 2019 recorded 48 617 new cases of lung cancer, of which 24912 died of this disease, making lung cancer the second leading cause of death in the country, only preceded by cardiovascular diseases.[10]

In the case of Guantánamo province, in 2022, 969 deaths were registered for lung carcinoma, and it is the second cause of death, in this sense, a behavior similar to that of the country is evidenced. The highest incidences are in the municipality of Guantánamo, in the South popular council [10].

For this reason, it is necessary to characterize the necrotic deceased with a clinical pathological diagnosis of lung carcinoma in the General Teaching Hospital during the study period in order to facilitate knowledge, guide diagnostic procedures and provide active follow-up, with the intention of favoring the quality of life of people with cancer through actions that facilitate the accessibility of medical care.

The presentation of lung carcinoma is not only a health problem, but also a social and economic problem.

The author's experience as a resident of the specialty of Pathological Anatomy of the General Teaching Hospital "Dr. Agusthino Neto" of Guantánamo, has allowed her to carry out empirical research during the exercise of her profession, as well as the systematization carried out on the subject, which shows that there are insufficiencies related to:

Late diagnosis of patients with lung cancer, which has an impact on the high mortality rate due to this disease.

Inadequacies in taking the clinical history with a comprehensive approach to the patient.

Based on these problems, the following scientific problem arises: What are the clinicopathological characteristics of the necrotic deceased with lung carcinoma at the General Teaching Hospital "Dr. Agostinho Neto" in the period from 2017 to 2020?

OBJECTIVES

General:

- To characterize necrotic decedents with a clinicopathological diagnosis of lung carcinoma at the General Teaching Hospital in the period 2017-2020.

Specific:

- To identify the sociodemographic factors present in the studied deceased.
- Determine the most frequent histologic type.
- To analyze the relationship between clinical stage and histologic type.

THEORETICAL FOUNDATIONS OF THE RESEARCH

Definition of lung carcinoma.

It is the malignant tumor of epithelial origin located in bronchi, bronchioles and alveoli, whose growth exceeds that of normal tissues and is not coordinated with it, it persists after the cessation of the stimuli that gave rise to it.

Epidemiology of lung carcinoma.

Carcinoma of the lung occurs mainly in older people. Most people diagnosed are 65 years of age or older; a very small number of people are younger than 45 years of age.

The average age of people at the time of diagnosis is approximately 70 years. It is diagnosed more in men than in women, although in recent years the diagnosis of this disease has increased in women (4).

The development of cancer involves the presence of several genetic alterations in the cell; a single alteration is not sufficient to cause cancer. These mutations accumulate in somatic cells throughout life, so that the probability of developing cancer, in most cases, increases considerably with age. (4)

In lung carcinoma there have been a series of epidemiological changes in recent decades. The frequency of carcinoma associated with tobacco (squamous cell carcinoma and small cell carcinoma) has decreased, and adenocarcinomas, which are not associated with this harmful element, have increased significantly in the female population, which is linked to genetic mutations discovered in recent years (5).

Etiology of lung carcinoma

Etiological factors of lung carcinoma include tobacco use, family or personal history of lung cancer. Harmful use of alcohol, obesity, low intake of fruits and vegetables and lack of physical activity [(7)].

The relationship with tobacco consumption depends mainly on the amount of daily consumption, the tendency to inhale smoke and the duration of smoking.

Smokers develop atypical alterations and epithelial hyperplasias. Among the carcinogenic substances that have been found in tobacco smoke are: (polycyclic aromatic hydrocarbons such as benzo pyrene) and promoting agents such as phenol derivatives. Radioactive elements such as: (polonium-210, carbon-14, potassium-40) and other contaminants such as arsenic, nickel, molds and additives have also been found.

Industrial hazards are another etiological factor of lung carcinoma. Radiation, uranium, asbestos, nickel, chromates, coal, gas, mustard, arsenic, beryllium and iron, newspaper workers, gold mines and people working with halo ether are less frequent etiological factors, but in general they do have a very negative influence on people who are exposed to them, atmospheric contamination by radon, especially in closed premises or in homes located where this product exists in the soil. [(11)]

Occasional observation of family groups suggests that there is a genetic predisposition, since in each of the generations this disease occurs even in the apparent absence of the influence of external risk factors.

Sometimes lung carcinoma is located in the vicinity of a scar and is called scar cancer, these tumors are mainly associated with scars produced in areas of old infarcts, metal foreign bodies, wounds and granulomatous infections such as tuberculosis [(12)].

Classification of lung carcinoma.

In general, in lung carcinoma as in other malignant neoplasms, histomorphological classifications are integrated with biological (genetic, molecular and immunophenotypic) and clinical knowledge to develop classifications that make practical sense, allowing prediction of clinical evolution and personalized, effective and curative treatment.

History of lung carcinoma:

One of the first classifications of lung carcinoma was proposed by Marchesani in 1924. It divided lung cancer into four main types, one of which was ciliated cell adenocarcinoma. This classification was in force for 25 years, but after the Second World War, the frequency of lung cancer increased notably and it became a public health problem. [(13)]

In 1967, the World Health Organization (WHO) published its first classification, after a broad consensus among expert pathologists, in which they considered the following types: Epidermoid carcinoma, Anaplastic small cell carcinoma, Adenocarcinoma, with the subtypes bronchogenic, acinar, papillary and bronchioloalveolar, Anaplastic large cell carcinoma, with the subtypes solid with mucin, solid without mucin, giant cell and clear cell and the combined(epidermoid carcinoma and adenocarcinoma).

It should be noted that this classification was based mainly on morphological aspects of the neoplasms, although also on anatomical locations and clinical course.

In 1981, the WHO published a new classification, based on the previous one, but with some modifications. Among the epithelial tumors, 8 main types were considered (squamous carcinoma, adenocarcinoma, small cell carcinoma and large cell carcinoma) and 70 pseudotumors of the pleura or lung were also described. Already in this classification the relationship between the clinical course and the main histological types is recognized [(14)]

In 2004, after a consensus meeting in Lyon, the WHO, in consensus with the IASLC (International Association for the Study of Lunch Cancer), published an official classification, on this occasion emphasizing the histological criteria for epithelial neoplasms, although the importance of auxiliary examinations in pathology was recognized[(15)].

The 2004 WHO classification defines the following malignant epithelial neoplasms:

- Squamous cell carcinoma and its variants (papillary, clear cell, small cell, basaloid).
- Small cell carcinoma and its combined variant.
- Adenocarcinoma and its types (acinar, papillary, bronchioloalveolar, mucinous and nonmucinous, mixed, solid with mucin production, various variants).

- Large cell carcinoma and its variants (neuroendocrine, combined, basaloid, lymphoepithelioma type, clear cell with rhabdoid phenotype).
- Adenosquamous carcinoma.
- Sarcomatoid carcinoma and its types (pleomorphic, spindle cell, giant cell, carcinosarcoma, pulmonary blastoma).
- Carcinoid Tumor (Typical and atypical)
- Type of salivary glands (mucoepidermoid, cystic adenoid, epithelial-myoepithelial)

Regarding pre-invasive lesions, atypical adenomatous hyperplasia (AAH) was defined as a localized proliferation of alveolar cells with mild to moderate atypia, without inflammation or fibrosis and with a characteristic ground-glass radiological image. Atypical endocrine cell hyperplasia (DIPNECH) was defined as the presence of small multifocal proliferations of neuroendocrine cells in the bronchiolar or bronchioloalveolar epithelium, with possible involvement of the adjacent interstitium. (15)

Basis for WHO classification of lung carcinoma in 2015.

Given the significant and rapid progress in the knowledge of the genetic and molecular mechanisms in the pathogenesis of lung cancer and their great relevance in the treatment of this disease, the WHO proposed a revision of the classification, especially in relation to adenocarcinoma.

Three societies sponsored this review, the ASLC, ERS and the ATS, the group of researchers was led by William D Travis, Elizabeth Brambilla and Masayuqui Noguchi. The recommendations were made according to the following topics ([16])

Molecular findings. The identification of mutations, translocations and other genetic alterations that are for subgroups of lung carcinomas (generally adenocarcinoma) has allowed the design of targeted therapies with successful responses. The altered genes include EGFR, KRAS, ALK, ROS, ERB2, BRAF, MET, etc. and are the current basis for molecular classification of lung carcinomas for the purpose of targeted therapies. This classification does not replace histological classification, but rather enriches it.

2. Small or cytologic samples. These are based on the importance of defining a diagnosis between adenocarcinoma or squamous carcinoma, since in the first case there may be responses to tyrosine kinase inhibitors (TKI) or to certain drugs such as pemetexed and in the second case there may be great toxicity by agents such as bevacizumab. For this the use of immunohistochemistry (IHQ) markers is recommended, although in a limited way (TTF1 AND NAPSIN-A for adenocarcinoma and P40 for squamous carcinoma). The recommendations are as follows:

For small or cytologic specimens, it is recommended that non-small cell lung carcinomas (NSCLC) be classified as adenocarcinoma or squamous cell carcinoma to the extent possible. In these cases, it is recommended that the term NSCLC be very limited and only used when it has not been possible to reach a specific diagnosis by morphology or IHC.

3. Recommendations for adenocarcinoma. The following recommendations were made: not to use the term bronchioloalveolar, because its diagnostic criteria correspond to adenocarcinoma in situ (AIS), an adequate denomination for these lesions. For solitary adenocarcinomas with a pure lipid pattern (formerly BAC) larger than 3 cm, the term AIS is recommended.

Complete surgical resection of these lesions is 100% curative. The vast majority of AIS are non-mucinous. For focal solitary adenocarcinoma (larger than 3 cm), with predominant lipid pattern and microscopic invasive foci of 0.5 cm or less, the new term minimally invasive adenocarcinoma (MIA) is recommended.

These patients have close to 100% disease-free survival if complete resection of the neoplasm is performed. Most of these tumors are non-mucinous.

For invasive adenocarcinoma, it is suggested to subtype according to their histologic patterns, in a semi-quantitative manner, in 5% increment and choose a single predominant pattern. It is recommended that the percentage of subtypes be reported.

In patients with multiple adenocarcinomas, histologic subtyping is suggested in comparison with the heterogeneous complex sample of histologic patterns to determine whether the tumor is metastatic or an isolated, metachronous or synchronous primary. For nonmucinous adenocarcinoma, previously classified as mixed subtype, in which the predominant subtype consists of a formerly termed nonmucinous BAC, it is recommended to use the term predominantly lipid adenocarcinoma and discontinue the term, mixed subtype.

In early adenocarcinoma, it is recommended to add predominantly micropapillary adenocarcinoma as a major subtype, when this is the case, since it has a poor prognosis. For adenocarcinomas previously classified as mucinous BAC, it is recommended to separate it from the adenocarcinoma previously called non-mucinous BAC and, depending on the extent of growth, lipidic or invasive, to classify them as mucinous AIS, mucinous MIA or for overtly invasive tumors, invasive adenocarcinoma.

According to the above, adenocarcinoma in situ is defined as a lesion in which the only growth pattern of tumor cells is along the alveolar walls, without invasion into the interstitium. The other growth patterns are those related to invasive adenocarcinoma, which maintain the three WHO 2004 classification patterns (acinar, papillary, solid) but adds, as already mentioned , micropapillary. A large proportion of resected adenocarcinomas show at least two different patterns.

The new classification recognizes the enteric subtype, with histomorphologic and immunohistochemical features similar to the intestinal primary, and the signet ring and clear cell types have been discarded, as they correspond more to cytologic variants that can be seen in adenocarcinoma subtypes. (17)

1. Squamous cell carcinoma.

In this type of carcinoma, the subtypes considered in the previous classification (papillary, clear cell and small cell) have been discarded because of their low clinical relevance and the difficulties in defining them adequately.

The basaloid type is maintained due to its unfavorable prognostic impact. Although they are not frequent, some molecular alterations have been identified that could be relevant for targeted therapy such as amplification of FGFR1 (20% of cases) and PI3K (8%), mutations of DDR2 (3%) and FGFR3 (1%). The importance of the use of IHC to differentiate it from adenocarcinoma in poorly differentiated cases (P40, TTF1, NAPSIN-A) has been emphasized for the reasons already stated.

2. Neuroendocrine tumors.

Given the clinical, epidemiological, molecular and genetic differences between carcinoid tumors and neuroendocrine carcinomas, these neoplasms are kept separate. Two types of neuroendocrine carcinoma are considered : small cell and large cell.

Although both have certain molecular and epidemiological similarities, it is not yet justified to integrate them into a single entity. Diffuse idiopathic pulmonary neuroendocrine cell hyperplasia is described as a pre-invasive lesion.

3. Large cell carcinoma and sarcomatoid carcinoma.

Large cell carcinoma loses morphologic and immunophenotypic differentiation of squamous or glandular lineage, so that it corresponds to an undifferentiated carcinoma. Sarcomatoid carcinoma is a generic term that encompasses pleomorphic, spindle cell, giant cell, carcinosarcoma and pulmonary blastoma carcinomas.

4. NUT carcinoma.

This rare carcinoma corresponds to a poorly differentiated neoplasm associated with a chromosomal rearrangement in the NUT gene. It is a translocation between this gene (NUTM1), located on chromosome 15p14 and other genes such as BDR4 and BDR3. It occurs at all ages, but more frequently in children or young adults.

Current WHO 2015 classification of lung carcinoma (adenocarcinoma).

Epithelial malignant neoplasm with glandular differentiation.[18)]

a. Lepidic: constituted by type II pneumocytes. It grows along the surface of the alveolar walls, with invasive areas of more than 5mm.

b. Acinar: glandular structure with central lumen surrounded by tumor cells.

c. Papillary: papillary growth of glandular neoplastic cells along a fibrovascular core.

d. Micropapillary: growth in small papillary nests without fibrovascular core.

e. Solid: predominant pattern with no evidence of lepidic, acinar, papillary or micropapillary pattern. If the solid pattern is 100%, there must be at least 5 or more mucin-producing cells per two high power fields, proven by histochemical staining.

f. Invasive mucinous: corresponds to the previously named mucinous BAC with columnar or goblet cell morphology with abundant intracytoplasmic mucin. In addition to the lepidic pattern, it can also present with other patterns.

g. Colloid: shows abundant mucin replacing the air spaces.

h. Fetal: histological structure similar to fetal lung tissue. It can be of high or low grade type.

i. Enteric: histological structure similar to colorectal adenocarcinoma.

j. Minimally invasive adenocarcinoma: Solitary adenocarcinoma, equal or smaller than 3cm in size, with a lepidic pattern, predominantly non mucinous and with invasion of up to 5mm in maximum dimension.

k. Preinvasive lesions: atypical adenomatous hyperplasia: localized atypical proliferation of type II pneumocytes or clear cells, up to 0.5 cm in maximal dimension.

Adenocarcinoma in situ: localized adenocarcinoma, usually non-mucinous, up to 3 cm in maximum dimension, growing along pre-existing alveolar structures, in a pure lepidic pattern, without stromal or vascular invasion.

Prognostic factors in lung carcinoma.

It includes location, tumor diameter, the presence or absence of regional and distant metastases and the clinical stage at which the diagnosis, resectability and administration of chemotherapy is made.[(19)]

Histology of lung carcinoma.

Histological characteristics are according to histogenesis and cellular differentiation: [3]

- Squamous carcinoma. Formation of horny globules, presence of intercellular bridges and individual cellular keratinization, characteristic of anaplasia with frequent atypical mitoses. They metastasize to lymph nodes, brain, lung, liver, etc. It is the variety most associated with smoking.
- Small cell undifferentiated carcinoma: It is characterized by the presence of lymphocytoid, spindle-shaped cells and in some cases large polygonal cells.
- Adenocarcinoma. It is characterized by the formation of glandular structures with different degrees of differentiation. Other varieties can be observed with formation of papillae, which are the papillary ones, and with muco secretion, which are the mucin-producing ones.

Undifferentiated large cell carcinomas often arise from a squamous carcinoma or adenocarcinoma that has become undifferentiated, in which the presence of large and giant cells is observed.

Staging of lung carcinoma.

Non-small cell lung cancer is classified into several stages following a rather complex system known by the acronym TNM. This makes it possible, firstly, to distinguish curable patients from those who are not curable and, secondly, to calculate the probability of being cured. [(20)]

T refers to the size of the tumor. Tx (positive cytology in bronchial secretions but not observable on CXR, CT or bronchoscopy) It is classified between T1 and T4, depending on whether the tumor is more voluminous or involves important nearby structures such as the main bronchi, arteries or heart.

- T0 No evidence of primary tumor.
- Tis: Carcinoma in situ.
- T1: Tumor 3 cm or less in greatest diameter, surrounded by lung or visceral pleura, and without bronchoscopic evidence of invasion more proximal than the lobar bronchus.
- T2: Tumor with any of the following in relation to size or extension: (greater than 3 cm in greatest diameter, involves the main bronchus 2 cm or more from the main carina, invades the visceral pleura, associated with atelectasis or obstructive pneumonitis extending to the hilar region but does not involve an entire lung).
- T3: Tumor of any size that directly invades any of the following: chest wall (includes tumors of the superior sulcus), diaphragm, mediastinal pleura or parietal pericardium; or tumor in the main bronchus within 2 cm of the main carina (1), but without involvement of the main carina; or atelectasis or associated obstructive pneumonitis of the whole lung.
- T4: Tumor of any size invading any of the following: mediastinum, heart, great vessels, trachea, esophagus, vertebral body, carina; tumor nodule/s separate from the original in the same lobe; tumor with malignant pleural effusion.

N indicates whether or not nearby nodes are affected. Nx (Minimum requirements for access to regional nodes are not met) (N0) means they are not. Node involvement is a very important prognostic factor that is graded from N1 to N3. To know if the most central lymph nodes of the thorax, in the mediastinal region, are invaded or not. Generally, mediastinal involvement means that the tumor is inoperable.

- N0: No regional lymph node metastases.
- N1: Metastases in ipsilateral peribronchial and/or hilar nodes, including direct extension.
- N2: Metastases in ipsilateral mediastinal and/or subcarinal nodes.
- N3: Metastases in contralateral mediastinal, contralateral hilar, scalene or supraclavicular nodes (ipsi or contralateral).

M indicates the presence or absence of metastases.

- MX: The presence of distant metastases cannot be assessed.
- M0: No distant metastasis.
- M1: Distant metastasis including tumor nodule/s in a different contralateral ipsio lobe.

Stadium classification

- Hidden Tx N0 M0
- Stadium 0 Tis N0 M0
- Stage IA T1 N0 M0

- Stage IB T2 N0 M0
- Stage IIA T1 N1 N1 M0
- Stage IIB T2 N1 M0 / T3 N0 M0
- Stage IIIA T1-3 N2 M0 / T3 N1 M0
- Stage IIIB T4 N0-3 M0 / T1-3 N3 M0
- Stage IV T1-4 N0-3 M1.

The rare superficial tumor of any size with the invasive component limited to the bronchial wall, which may extend proximally to the main bronchus, is also classified as T1.

Most pleural effusions associated with lung cancer are due to tumor. However, there are some patients in whom multiple cytopathologic studies of pleural fluid are negative for tumor.

In these cases, the fluid is not hematic and is not an exudate. When these elements and clinical judgment indicate that the effusion is not related to the tumor, the effusion should be excluded as a classification element, and the patient should be considered as T1, T2 or T3.

The great vessels (T4) are: Aorta, superior vena cava, inferior vena cava, pulmonary artery trunk, intrapericardial segments of right or left pulmonary artery trunk, intrapericardial segments superior or inferior pulmonary veins, right or left.

Additional comments on clinical classification (pre-thoracotomy) (AJCC-UICC-1993; SEPAR-1998)

Patients with a malignant pleural effusion, i.e., cytology positive for cancer or clinically related to the underlying neoplasm are coded as T4.

Pericardial effusion is classified in the same way as pleural effusion. Direct involvement of the parietal pericardium is classified T3; involvement of the visceral pericardium, T4.

Vocal cord paralysis (resulting from involvement of the recurricular branch of the vagus nerve), superior vena cava obstruction, or compression of the trachea or esophagus may be related to direct extension of the primary tumor or nodal involvement. The therapeutic options and prognosis associated with these manifestations of disease extension fall into the T4-stage IIIb category; therefore, a T4 classification is recommended. If the primary tumor is peripheral and clearly unrelated to vocal cord paralysis, superior vena cava obstruction, or compression of the trachea and esophagus, then nodal classification according to established rules is appropriate.

Invasion of the phrenic nerve, which invariably indicates direct extension of the primary tumor, is classified as T3. Pleural tumor foci that are not in continuity with the primary tumor should be considered as T4.

A discontinuous lesion outside the parietal pleura in the chest wall or diaphragm should be considered as M1. Peripheral tumors that directly invade the chest wall and ribs are classified as T3.

METHODOLOGICAL DESIGN

Type of study: In order to achieve the proposed research objectives, a retrospective cross-sectional descriptive study was carried out.

Population and sample

The study population represents the set of individuals that we wish to study and that meet certain characteristics. The study sample is the subset of the population being studied with particular characteristics, in order to draw conclusions from that population.

The population consisted of 155 deceased with a diagnosis of lung carcinoma at necropsy, the sample was selected by non-probabilistic purposive sampling, taking into account the inclusion and exclusion criteria, and consisted of 114 deceased necropsied with a histological diagnosis of lung carcinoma before death.

Inclusion criteria

- Deceased with carcinoma of the lung necropsied at HGD
- That the death occurred in the period from January 2017 through December 2020.
- Histological diagnosis of lung carcinoma before death.

Exclusion criteria

- Deceased with carcinoma of the lung that has not been necrotized.
- Documentation that does not contain all the data necessary for the investigation.

- Deceased with a diagnosis of secondary or metastatic lung carcinoma.

Operationalization of variables.

Variables constitute the different forms or manifestations of a certain characteristic or phenomenon"; in the context of research, a variable is a fact, a phenomenon that can assume different forms, manifestations or values.

The variables were operationalized as follows:

- Age group variable: discrete, independent, quantitative variable. It is an age range or set, formed by people who share the same age or vital moment, which are of statistical or academic interest. Calculating the years from the date of birth

Classification scale: Intercalar. Operationalized in three groups

- Group 1. From 20 years old to 50 years old
- Group 2. From 51 years old to 81 years old
- Group 3. Over 81 years old

Final expression of the variable: It is considered according to the date of birth described in the medical record.

- Variable: socio-demographic characteristics: qualitative, nominal, discrete polytomous, independent. These are the general characteristics of a population group. These traits shape the identity of the members of this group.

The variables were operationalized as follows: residence (urban or rural), smoking habit (yes or no), family history of lung carcinoma (yes or no), occupation (worker, student, retired, housewife or unemployed).

1. Residence (qualitative nominal dichotomous discrete dichotomous qualitative, independent)

- Categories: urban, rural.

  ✓ Urban: are those where the city, large towns or metropolitan areas are located. The population density is higher, with a minimum of 2,500 inhabitants and is characterized by the development of a diverse economy, focused on the secondary and tertiary sectors.

  ✓ Rural: adjective used to indicate that which is related to the countryside and agricultural and livestock workers. It is characterized by having fewer inhabitants in comparison with its geographical space, which is usually larger. Development of the primary economy.

Final expression of the variable: place where they resided at the time of diagnosis.

2. Smoking habit: Qualitative, discrete, independent, dichotomous, nominal, discrete dichotomous. It is the usual consumption of any tobacco product. It is a behavior learned by the individual.

- Categories: yes, no.

Final expression of the variable: it is considered whether the patient was a smoker or not at the time of diagnosis.

3. APF of lung cancer Qualitative nominal dichotomous discrete dichotomous, independent)

It is the registration of lung carcinoma in biological relatives of an individual, both living and dead. It is the genetic predisposition or susceptibility that influences the phenotype of an individual organism, or of a particular species.

- Categories: yes, no.

Final expression of the variable: the presence or absence of the variable as described in the clinical history is considered.

4. Occupation: qualitative qualitative nominal discrete polytomous, independent.

It is the type or type of work performed with job specification.

- Categories: (Worker, student, retired, housewife or unemployed).
  - ✓ Worker: a natural person who performs subordinate personal work for another natural or legal person.
  - ✓ Student: a person who is studying in an educational institution.
  - ✓ Retiree: a person who has reached retirement status.
  - ✓ Housewife: is the person whose main occupation is the home, dedicating herself to reproductive work as well as to unpaid housework.
  - ✓ Unoccupied: a person who is inactive. That is empty of things or free to be employed by someone.

Final expression of the variable: the presence or absence of the variable as described in the clinical history is considered.

- Variable Histologic type (qualitative nominal discrete polytomous qualitative, independent).

It is the identification of a disease by examining cells or tissues under a microscope.

The variables were operationalized as follows:

- Categories:

  ✓ squamous cell carcinoma

  ✓ adenocarcinoma

  ✓ small cell carcinoma

  ✓ large cell carcinoma

  ✓ adenosquamous carcinoma (mixed)

  ✓ sarcomatoid carcinoma

  ✓ carcinoid tumor

Final expression of the variable: it is considered as described in the clinical history and necropsy protocol.

- Variable clinical stage of lung carcinoma. Qualitative, discrete, independent, polytomous, nominal.

It is the period or phases of development of a malignant lesion in an individual, with its own characteristics, which differentiate it from the other periods of development.

- Categories:
  - ✓ Tumor
  - ✓ regional lymph nodes
  - ✓ distant metastases.

The variables were operationalized as follows:

- Categories: I, II, III, IV

Final variable expression: According to TNM classification. It is considered as described in the clinical history.

Ethical aspects

The names of the patients, their initials, and the numbers assigned to them at necropsy were not included, in order to protect the confidentiality of the information. The information has been used only for scientific purposes.

Stages of the investigation:

The research was divided into two stages, the diagnostic or information gathering stage and the final evaluation stage.

Diagnostic stage: To carry out this first stage, authorization was requested from the head of the Anatomic Pathology department to access the necropsy protocols for the years included in the study and to obtain the study population and sample, and from the head of the archive department to collect the information from the medical records.

Final evaluation stage

The primary data collected and recorded in tables and graphs were distributed according to the operationalization of the variables proposed above, the results were evaluated, analyzed and discussed, and conclusions were reached.

Methods

Empirical methods

- Documentary analysis: a review of the clinical histories, the cancer registry and the registry of deceased persons was carried out in order to obtain the necessary data for the research.

Theoretical methods

- Historical-logical for the analysis of specialized literature and documentation, with the objective of examining the historical background that characterizes the object of study up to the present day.
- Deductive-inductive: to infer from the results obtained from the research, as well as to regroup all the information obtained and specify the current state of the problem and its behavior.
- Analysis and synthesis: allowed the influence of each variable to be studied.

Techniques and procedures

Technique for obtaining information

At the "Dr. Agostinho Neto" General Teaching Hospital, an analysis of the necessary documents (clinical histories and autopsy reports) and an extensive and updated review of the subject in the electronic network available to health professionals (Infomed), Google Scholar and the available bibliography were carried out.

Subsequently, data were collected from each personal file according to the previously prepared emptying form and the operationalization of the variables, in order to obtain the primary data.

Analysis and processing techniques

All the data collected were transferred to a record sheet and the survey was used as a guide for the collection of information.

It was used as a summary measure of quantitative variables in number and percentage.

Analysis and processing

The information collected through this study has nominal variables grouped into categories, if possible mutually exclusive, for appropriate presentation in tabular or graphical form.

The means of analysis used were those determined by descriptive statistics. These data were presented in graphic tables, discussed by comparing them with the results of other authors published in the bibliographic references, which were obtained through electronic search, aided by computer techniques (electronic journals, MEDLINE, LILACS, GOOGLE, HINARIS, etc.), processed by means of Microsoft Word and Epi info programs. Conclusions were reached and recommendations were issued.

ANALYSIS AND DISCUSSION OF RESULTS

Lung carcinoma is a serious health problem and a leading cause of mortality worldwide. Although the disease is often considered a first world problem, in reality more than half of all malignant tumors are reported in developing countries, where the resources available for prevention, diagnosis and treatment are limited.

Lung carcinoma is currently the third most common type of cancer and the leading cause of death in the Americas, with 324,000 new cases and nearly 262,000 deaths each year. In the male population, the highest incidence and mortality rates are recorded in countries such as Uruguay, the United States and Cuba, and the lowest in Central America and Bolivia. According to projections, by the year 2030 there will be more than 541,000 new cases and around 445,000 deaths from lung cancer in the Americas.[(21]

Distribution according to age group.

Lung carcinoma occurs mainly in older people. Most people diagnosed with lung carcinoma are 65 years of age or older; a very small number of people are younger than 45 years of age. The average age of people at the time of diagnosis is approximately 70 years, figures reported by the WHO and consistent with most countries. [(21)]

Table 1. Distribution according to age group. Clinicopathological characterization of deceased necrotic patients with lung carcinoma at the Hospital General Docente Agustino Neto.2017-2020.

Age group	Number	%
Group 1(20-50)	4	3.5
Group 2(51-81)	63	55.3
Group 3(+ 81)	47	41.2
Total	114	100

Source: Necropsy protocols.

In this study, the age group with the highest number of deaths was between 51 and 81 years with 63 deaths for 55.3%, followed by the age group over 81 years with 47 deaths for 41.2%. (Table 1)

According to UNEO estimates for 2019, the population aged 65 years or older will account for 11.6% of the total and the population aged 60 years or older for 16.3%, making Cuba the second most aged country in Latin America after Uruguay. At the same time, over the decades, there has been a gradual decrease in the population between 0 and 14 years of age, which represents 18.2%. The average age of the population is 37.3 years, with about 38 years for women and 36.6 for men [(22)]

Recent studies have confirmed that by the year 2025, the island will be the most aged country in the region and one of the 25 most aged countries in the world. In the region, Cuba, together with Argentina,

Chile and Uruguay, belongs to the group of countries with an advanced demographic transition , characterized by populations with moderate or low birth and mortality rates, which translates into a low natural growth rate of around 1%.[22]

In Cuba cancer constitutes one of the most relevant problems for public health.In the period studied malignant tumors were the second cause of death in Cuba in all ages, in the year 2017 with 25232 cases with a rate of 224.4%, figures that were increasing until the year 2020 presented figures of 26289 cases for a rate of 234.7%, with predominance always in the age group older than 40 years. With much higher figures in the case of those over 60 years of age, with 19894 people. [9]

Similar behavior is presented in the province of Guantánamo where malignant tumors are the second cause of death in the period under study with an average of 866 cases for a rate of 22.41%, with a predominance in the age group over 40 years old and specifically those over 60 years old with 681 cases for a rate of 78.63%.

The most frequently diagnosed cancers in men are prostate (21.7%), lung (9.5%) and colorectal (8.0%). In women, the most frequent cancers are breast (25.2%), lung (8.5%) and colorectal (8.2%), but lung carcinoma is the one with the highest mortality rate. [9,10]

Dr. Roberto Gonzales, from the Public Health System Hospital in Chile, which conducted a descriptive study of characterization, staging and survival in deceased with lung cancer between 2010 and 2019, in which the largest number of its sample studied in the distribution by age were those over 61 years old with 61.4%. [23]

Dr. Adriana Cabo García y colectivo, of the general teaching hospital" Dr. Juan Bruno Zayas Alfonso, of Santiago de Cuba", conducted a descriptive study on Clinical and epidemiological aspects in patients with lung cancer of 125 patients, in the period 2015 to 2016 and in that study the largest number of patients were from the age group between 51-69 years (90 patients for 72.0%) [(24)]

In the study conducted by Odalis machandi Thomas, on the demographic characterization of the province of Guantanamo from 2013 to 2017, it was evidenced that the province of guantanamo has more than 15% of the population aged 60 years and over, with respect to the total.[(25)]

When analyzing the above information, it can be highlighted that the risk of lung carcinoma increases with increasing age, which is very important, given the aging of the current population, which coincides with the increase in the diagnosis of lung carcinoma and its high mortality in the period under study.

Distribution according to socio-demographic characteristics.

Sociodemographic characteristics are the general characteristics of a population group. These traits shape the identity of the members of this population group.

The sociodemographic study allows to know the structure and dynamics of a population, as well as to identify the necessary resources for the projections of development plans and future actions that enhance the welfare of the population in a given territory. It is therefore essential to study the demographic variables to characterize the sample studied and to determine the interrelationship between it and its own development.

Table 2. DISTRIBUTION according to socio-demographic characteristics.

		Number	Percent
Residence	Rural	18	15.8
	Urbana	96	84.2
Smoking habit	Yes	8	7.0
	No	106	93
APF of lung carcinoma	Yes	10	8.8
	No	104	91.2
Occupation	Worker	77	67.51
	Retired	28	24.6
	Student	--	--
	Housewife	7	6.14
	Unemployed	2	1.75

Source: Medical records.

This study analyzed the behavior of sociodemographic variables (Residence, smoking habits, family pathological history of lung carcinoma and occupation) in the necrotized deceased at the General Teaching Hospital, in the period 2017 to 2020 with lung carcinoma already diagnosed before their death and their relationship between them.

Residence

The country's population is distributed in cities and towns of urban character; the provinces with the lowest urbanity indexes are Las Tunas (62.2 %) and Guantánamo (60.5 %), and while 100 % of the population of Havana province is urban, followed by Matanzas with 82.2 %. Maisí municipality is the most rural 91.59 % in 2019. [10]

It was observed in this study that 84.2% of the deceased with lung carcinoma were from urban areas (Guantánamo municipality) and only 15.8% were from rural areas (Table 2). The period under study in Cuba coincides with the highest incidence of deaths in urban areas with 88174 cases for a rate of 83.03% and with the number of inhabitants in the urban area of the province of Guantánamo.[9]

In spite of the percentage of urban population, the rural population is distributed in practically all the municipalities, and is concentrated in some that conform spaces of particular interest. There are 32 (19%) municipalities with more than 50% of their population in rural areas, and as a historical characteristic, the greatest concentration of them is found in the mountainous eastern provinces, Guantánamo, Granma and Santiago de Cuba, in that order.[9,10]

However, very high percentages of rural population are found in municipalities in the plains of the western and central-eastern part of the country. Examples of these are the contiguous tobacco-growing municipalities of extreme south-western part of the island of Cuba, San Juan y Martínez and San Luis with 65.46% and 75.74% of rural population respectively, and the also contiguous municipalities of Najasa with 78.95% and Jimaguayú with 83.70% in the province of Camagüey. [9,10]

Taking into account the information published in the Guantánamo Statistical Yearbook of 2019, the population in the period studied was 227112 on average and its distribution according to place of residence were 110074.8 in the urban area and 8778 in the rural area on average, being evident that the largest population according to territorial distribution in the province of Guantánamo is found in the urban area in the period studied. (9)

Alexei Santana Galano, Dr. Soraya Teherán Plumier, among others, conducted a study on cancer mortality in the adult population of Baracoa, in 4234 patients, where lung cancer continues to be the most lethal neoplasm in the period from 2001 to 2010, also significantly affecting intermediate adults (26).

Dr. Alfredo Rousseaux Modesí, Leonel Blanco García and others, conducted a research study on mortality from malignant tumors in the 4 de Abril polyclinic, in the municipality of Guantánamo in 2013, with the aim of characterizing the behavior of mortality from malignant tumors in that health area, with a population of 327 deceased and among the most frequent tumors were lung and prostate cancer, with necropsies performed and confirmed diagnoses. The majority were over 60 years of age, with a tendency to increase as the years went by during the period studied (27)

Smoking habit

Smoking is one of the main risk factors predisposing to lung carcinoma. In the United States, smoking is linked to 80 to 90% of deaths from lung carcinoma. The consumption of tobacco products, such as cigars and pipes, also increases the risk of developing lung carcinoma. (4)

The risk increases with increasing age and with the number of cigarettes smoked per day. Quitting smoking at any age decreases the risk of lung carcinoma.

Secondhand smoke and the harmful chemicals in cigarettes are known causes of cardiovascular disease, stroke and lung cancer in non-smoking adults.

It is necessary to point out that in the sample studied, the most affected were the deceased non-smokers, with a percentage of 93%, not coinciding with other investigations that were found, nor with those referred to in this text. This makes us reflect on which etiological and demographic factors are more notable in the study sample that predisposed to lung carcinoma (Table 2). (Table 2).

Cuba is the first per capita consumer of cigarettes in America, has a very high incidence rate in this habit, both for women and men, and in the case of women it compares with international figures. In general, 60% of men and 40% of women who smoke consume more than 20 cigarettes a day [(28)]

Dr. Adriana Cabo García, from the general teaching hospital "Dr. Juan Bruno Zayas Alfonso, Santiago de Cuba", conducted a study in which the largest number of patients were smokers, 122 for 97.6%, of whom 73.8% consumed more than 20 cigarettes a day and 89.3% had smoked for more than 30 years before diagnosis [(24)]

Family pathologic history of lung carcinoma

The role of hereditary factors is less well understood for lung cancer than for other cancers. Although there is no conclusive genetic alteration that defines lung cancer risk, numerous studies suggest that first-degree relatives have an increased risk of developing lung cancer.

The factors analyzed in this study, the most affected deceased were non-smokers and those with no family history of lung carcinoma, with a percentage of 93% and 91.2%, respectively.

A meta-analysis of 28 case-control studies and 17 observational cohort studies showed an increased risk of lung cancer associated with having an affected relative (relative risk 1.8, 95% CI 1.6-2.0). The risk was higher in family members with relatives diagnosed with lung cancer at an early age and with multiple affected family members.[29]

Other studies have found a lower but still significant risk of lung cancer in second and third degree relatives, especially when associated with other environmental factors, such as smoking, exposure to substances such as radon, and exposure to radiation that is carcinogenic. [9,10]

The above coincides with the study conducted by Dr. Ana Esther Jiménez Massa at the Salamanca Hospital, since the predominant risk factors were a first and second degree family history of lung cancer and also people with a history of having suffered from other types of cancer in previous years, most of whom were smokers or former smokers [30]

Dr. Adriana Cabo García, in her research on Clinical and epidemiological aspects in patients with lung cancer, 83 of the sample had a family history of lung cancer, 66.0%, while 34.0% had no family history of lung cancer, being first-degree relatives. [24]

This study does not coincide with the findings of the research cited above or with those published by the WHO, given that the sample studied was dominated by deceased persons with no family history of lung cancer and no history of smoking.

Occupation

The number of people working in Cuba increased in 2019, the favorable behavior of the previous year, when for the first time the "curve" rose after decreasing for three consecutive calendars. The increase was 102 520, much higher than in 2018 (just 7 900), as revealed by the National Statistics and Information Office (ONEI). [9,22]

This is good news, especially considering that those employed in the economy represent only 41% of the total population [10]

In the sample under study, there was a predominance of deceased workers with 77 cases (67.54%), followed by retirees with 28 cases (24.57%). (Table 2)

In addition to the strong tension imposed by the demographic dynamic itself, which is manifested in low fertility rates and high life expectancy, there are also those who, for various reasons, do not enter the workforce.

The figures published in the 2022 edition of the Statistical Yearbook of Cuba indicate growth in both the state and non-state sectors. An interesting fact is the number of workers hired by the State, which increases (11 547 more than those accounted for in 2018) after declining during the last few years.[10]

In Guantánamo, people of working age prevailed for a total of 142396.5 (including men aged 17-64 and women aged 17-59) and outside working age 84715.5 on average in the period under study. [10]

Occupational factors are the second most important cause of lung carcinoma. Several studies indicate that between 9 and 15% of these tumors diagnosed in men and around 5% of those in women can be attributed to the inhalation of carcinogenic substances in the work environment [31,32].

Among a large number of substances, asbestos is considered to be the most important occupational carcinogen. Exposure can be direct, in mines and industries (textiles, automobile workshops, cement, insulation, shipyards, etc.) or indirect, in the home, through impregnated clothing. [4]

It has been estimated for Spain that 4% of lung carcinomas are related to this mineral. The possibility of developing a tumor is linked, especially with the use of amphibole fibers, with the intensity and duration of exposure to asbestos. In addition, the risk is higher with concomitant exposure to tobacco smoke [33, 34]

The data analyzed above coincide with the sample in the period studied. In the province of Guantánamo there is presence of factories that although they are located in rural areas and others in the periphery of the city, they are located near very large populations, so the latter are exposed to carcinogenic substances such as radioactive minerals, inhaled chemicals such as arsenic, beryllium, cadmium, silica, vinyl chloride, nickel compounds, chromium compounds, coal products, diesel combustion products and radon.

In recent years, government and industry have taken steps to help protect workers from many of these exposures, but consideration must also be given to the population surrounding these institutions who are themselves exposed to the risks posed by these industries.

When analyzing these data as a whole (distribution according to socio-demographic characteristics) with respect to the distribution according to occupation and place of origin (Table 2), in which those who died with lung carcinoma from rural areas, workers and retirees had a high frequency, it is relevant to take into account risk factors in the work environment in urban areas that predispose or considerably influence the predisposition to lung carcinoma ( ).

Although in this study, it was not possible to be specific about the place or jobs performed by the deceased in the study, due to the absence of such data in the clinical history, it is very important to take into account the exposure to factors that predispose to lung carcinoma in urban workers, since they predominated in the study.

This makes us reflect on the sources of work in the city of Guantánamo and the harmful occupational factors that could influence the predisposition to lung carcinoma, among which the most frequent are MINSAP workers, education, lawyers, electricity, gas and water supply, construction, drivers, hotels and restaurants, economy and commerce, sports and culture, police, communal workers and account holders.

In the city, air pollution (especially near busy roads) appears to increase the risk of lung carcinoma, with some researchers estimating that globally about 5% of all lung carcinoma deaths may be due to outdoor air pollution and air contaminated by the combustion of diesel or other petroleum products released from vehicles in the city. [31,32]

Distribution according to histological type.

Cancer cells and tissue are characterized under the microscope according to histological characteristics, which allows for classification and gives an idea of how fast these cells could multiply and spread. This is done for diagnostic and/or prognostic purposes.

Distribution according to histologic type.

Histological types	**Number**	**%**
Squamous cell carcinoma	52	45.6
Adenocarcinoma	40	35.1
Small cell carcinoma	15	13.2
Large cell carcinoma	7	6.1
Total	114	100

Source: Medical records and necropsy protocols.

It was observed that in the study 45.6% of the deceased necrotic patients were diagnosed with squamous cell carcinoma, 35.1% with adenocarcinoma and only 6.1% with large cell carcinoma. This coincides with the majority of the studies found and discussed below.

According to the WHO, the most frequent lung carcinoma is non-small cell lung carcinoma with about 80 to 85% of the cases and between 10 to 15% are small cell lung carcinoma. [7]

Study conducted at the Hospital Nacional Sur Este in the state of Cusco in patients diagnosed with lung carcinoma, the most frequent histological types were Adenocarcinoma with 72.22% and small cell carcinoma was present in 5.5%.[35]

Study carried out at the Policlínico Universitario Fermín Valdez Domínguez of Viñales in 2022, the most frequent was non-small cell carcinoma with 61.54%, without specifying the histological type [36]

Dr. Adriana Cabo García y colectivo, of the general teaching hospital "Dr. Juan Bruno Zayas Alfonso, of Santiago de Cuba", in her research on Clinical and epidemiological aspects in patients with lung cancer, the most frequent histological type was lung adenocarcinoma [24]

Distribution according to clinical stage.

The clinical stage of lung carcinoma allows for quantification of disease aggressiveness, information sharing, surgical eligibility, treatment design, assessment of outcomes at the end of treatment, and disease follow-up. [20]

It is always considered on the basis of the cytohistological diagnosis. The TNM classification of malignant tumors describes the extent of the cancer in a patient's body. T describes the primary tumor. N describes the lymphatic regions and M describes the metastasis [20]

Table 4. Distribution according to clinical stage

Clinical stage	Number	%
II	5	4.4
III	100	87.7
IV	9	7.9
Total	114	100

Source: Medical records.

It was observed in the study that 87.7% of the deceased necrotized with lung carcinoma were diagnosed in stage III, 7.9% in stage IV and in stage I, no deceased was diagnosed.

Study conducted at the Hospital Nacional Sur Este in the state of Cusco in patients diagnosed with lung carcinoma, the most frequent clinical stage was stage IV at the time of diagnosis with 61.11% and 16.67% in stage III (35)

At the National Institute of Neoplastic Diseases in Lima, Peru, a study was conducted on lung cancer, a review of current knowledge, diagnostic methods and therapeutic perspectives in which the most frequent clinical stage was stage III and IV (37)

At the University Polyclinic Fermín Valdez Domínguez of Viñales, the characterization of patients with lung cancer was carried out. At the time of diagnosis, 42.31% were found in stage III with 22 cases and 32.69% in stage IV (36)

Dr. Adriana Cabo García y colectivo, of the "Dr. Juan Bruno Zayas Alfonso" General Teaching Hospital in Santiago de Cuba, conducted a descriptive study on clinical and epidemiological aspects in patients with lung cancer, a high percentage of which corresponded to stage IV of the disease (24)

In this regard, Dr. Luis Paz-Ares, head of the Medical Oncology Department at the Hospital 12 de Octubre (Madrid) and president of the Oncosur Foundation, explained the main problems associated with lung cancer: the high incidence and late diagnosis.

And with respect to this he expressed: "It is the most deadly tumor in the western world, almost 2 million people die from this cause, mainly associated with tobacco. It is important to start detecting it earlier, since if we were to diagnose all lung tumors at less than one centimeter, 90% of the cases would be cured".[6]

It is therefore necessary to create new strategies that favor the early diagnosis of lung cancer, in order to reduce mortality from this disease, which affects so many lives every year, despite the wide knowledge of the disease and its risk factors.

Distribution according to the relationship of the clinicopathological characteristics.

Relation of the clinical pathological characteristics is very necessary given the high frequency of cancerous diseases affecting the population and the increase in mortality due to this cause.

Therefore, the best way to face this disease is to join the efforts of all the professionals who work every day in its diagnosis and treatment.

Distribution according to clinical pathological relationship.

	Histological types									
Clinical stage	**Squamous cell carcinoma**		**Adenocarcinoma**		**Small cell carcinoma**		**Large cell carcinoma**		**No.**	**%**
	#	%	#	%	#	%	#	%		
II	3	2.6	--	--	2	1.8	--	--	5	4.4
III	48	42.1	36	31.6	13	11.4	3	2.6	100	87.7
IV	1	0.9	4	3.5	--	--	4	3.5	9	7.9
Total	52	45.6	40	35.1	15	13.2	7	6.1	114	100

Source: Medical records and necropsy protocols.

The relation of the pathological clinical characteristics facilitates the knowledge of special situations, specific plans are established, diagnostic procedures are oriented and active follow-up can be given. For this reason, its intention is to favor the quality of life of people with cancer through actions that facilitate the accessibility of medical assistance.

The study showed that clinical stage III was the most frequent in necrotic lung carcinoma deaths, corresponding to the histological types: squamous cell carcinoma with 42.1%, adenocarcinoma with 31.6% and only 4.4% were in clinical stage II, corresponding to the histological types: squamous cell carcinoma and small cell carcinoma with 2.6% and 1.8% respectively.

In order to study, diagnose and treat lung carcinoma, the combination of clinical features and anatomopathological diagnosis is of vital importance to offer the best results and thus apply timely treatment and improve the quality of life of patients and in other cases reduce or delay cancerous growth.

When lung carcinoma is diagnosed in clinical stage III, nearby lymph nodes are already invaded by the tumor, that is, it is a locally advanced tumor disease. The chances that it has spread are greater, which decreases the possibility that the tumor can be surgically removed and it may have to be treated with a combination of chemotherapy and radiation followed by immunotherapy, which influences the high mortality rate due to this disease. [(20)]

The drugs used for the treatment of lung carcinoma have benefits for the patient but can also produce adverse effects, in addition to decreasing survival, which is 5 years for 37% of patients diagnosed in stage III and 9% for those diagnosed in stage IV of the disease according to the American Cancer Association [(20)]

CONCLUSIONS

The necrotized deceased with lung carcinoma at the General Teaching Hospital "Dr. Agostinho Neto" in the period under study were characterized, taking into account age, sociodemographic factors, most frequent histological type and its relationship with the clinical stage at the time of diagnosis, drawing attention to the predominance of risk factors in the occupational setting, the histological type squamous cell carcinoma and its diagnosis in advanced stages of the disease, which favors the determination of common features in the study sample.

RECOMMENDATIONS

The results of the research show the need to implement new strategies to promote the early diagnosis of lung carcinoma in order to reduce mortality from this disease and thus improve the quality of life of patients, their families and the population in general, and undoubtedly have a positive influence on the country's economy.

BIBLIOGRAPHIC REFERENCES

1. Torres Vaca M, Zarco Villavicencio A, Peña Rodríguez S, López Hernández MA, Briones Quiroz MS. Manual for the exploration of pulmonary fields [Internet]. 1st ed. Mexico : Universidad Nacional Autónoma de México; 2022 [Cited 2024 Apr 19] Available at: https:

2. Castañeda C. Intestinal microbiota and the first 1000 days of life. Rev. Cuban Pediatr. [Internet]. 2021 [Cited July 3 2021]; 93(3):e1382. Available at: https://revpediatria.sld.cu/index.php/ped/article/view/1382/823

3. Castañeda C. The intestinal microbiota. Chapter 2. In: Human intestinal microbiota and its challenges. Quito: Ed. El Siglo; 2020. [cited 2020 Dec] Available from: http://scielo.sld.cu/scielo.php?script=sci_arttext&pid=S003475312021000400012

4. García-Rodríguez M, Benavides-Márquez A, Ramírez-Reyes E, Gallego-Escobar Y, Toledo-Cabarco Y, Chávez-Chacón M. Lung cancer: some epidemiological, diagnostic and treatment considerations. Camagüey Medical Archive [Internet]. 2018 [cited 19 Apr 2024]; 22 (5) :[approx. 11 p.]. Available from: https://revistaamc.sld.cu/index.php/amc/article/view/5610

5. World Health Organization. Histological typing of lung tumors! n.d. ed. Geneva: Kreyberg; 2020. [cited 2021 Dec] Available from: https:

6. Álvarez Matos Dunia, Nazario Dolz Ana María, Romero García Lázaro Ibrahim, Castillo Toledo Luis, Rodríguez Fernández Zenén, Miyares Peña María Victoria. Characterization of patients operated on

for non-small cell lung cancer. Rev Cubana Cir [Internet]. 2020 Jun [cited 2024 Apr 19] ; 59(2): e962. Available from: http:

7. PAHO/WHO.Cancer Country Profiles, 2020. . [cited 2020 Dec] Available from: https://www3.paho.org/hq/index.php?option=com_content&view=artc

8. Rodríguez Cruz AM. Lung cancer: first cause of death in Cuba. Juventud Rebelde [Internet]. 2020 [cited 20 December 2020];:1-2. Available from: https:

9. Ministry of Public Health. Health Statistical Yearbook. Havana, 2020. [cited 2021 Feb] Available from:

https://salud.msp.gob.cu/wp-content/Anuario/Anuario-2020.pdf

10. Ministry of Public Health. Health Statistical Yearbook. Havana, 2022. [cited 2023 Marz] Available at: https:

11. Caron Girón J, Cuellar López D, Beltrán González BM, Hernández Ruiz RA, Acebo Rodríguez M, Águila Curbelo Y. Characterization of lung cancer in adults according to clinical and epidemiological variables. Rev Medicen Electró [Cited 2024 Apr 19];*28*(1): 1-20 Available in: http:

12. Hernández Suarez N, Rabelo Dapino D, Sánchez Sandrino M, Rojas Morena B Hernández Díaz N. Clinical epidemiological characterization of lung cancer in patients attended. Rev. Cien Med Pinar del Río [Internet]. 2020 [Cited 2024 Apr 19]; 24(1):21-28. Available at: http://scielo.sld.cu/scielo.php?script=sci_arttext&pid=S1561-31942020000100021&lng=es.

13. The World Health Organization histological typing of lung tumours. Second edition. American journal of clinical pathology [Internet]. 1982 [Cited 2024 Apr 19]; 77(2): 123-136. Available at: https:

14. Travis WD, Brambilla E, Nicholson AG, Yatabe Y, Austin JHM, Beasley MB, et al;. World Health Organization. Histological typing of lung tumors. [Internet]. 2015 [Cited 2024 Apr 19]; 40(2): 90-7.] Available from:https://pubmed-ncbi-nlm-nihgov.translate.goog/?term=Beasley+MB&cauthor_id=26291008&_x_tr_sl=en&_x_tr_tl=en&_x_tr_hl=en&_x_tr_pto=sc

15. Barrionuevo Cornejo Carlos, Dueñas Hancco Daniela. Current classification of lung carcinoma. Histological, immunophenotypic, molecular and clinical considerations. Horiz. Med [Internet]. 2019 Oct [cited 2024 Apr 19]; 19(4):74-83. Available from: http:

16. Ciri6n G, Herrera M. Pathologic Anatomy: Topics for cytohistopathology. Havana: Ecimed. [Internet]. 2010 [Cited 2024 Apr 19]; Available from: http:

17. Ríos Hidalgo N. General Pathology [Internet]. 1st ed. Havana: Ecimed; 2014 [Cited 2024 Apr 19] Available at: https://www.google.es/url?sa=t&source=web&rct=j&opi=89978449&url=https://instituciones.sld.cu/inor/files/2023/03/Patolog%25C3%25ADa-general.pdf&ved=2ahUKEwj0tPHorM6FAxXNpLAFHURhDygQFnoECB4QAQ&usg=AOvVaw0p7bm5UUz8qGc8079aO6Ke

18. Hurtado de Mendoza Amat J. Autopsy. Quality assurance in medicine. [Internet]. 2nd ed. Havana: Editorial Ciencias Médicas; 2014. ch13 Annexes p. 183-185. Available at: http:

19. Sainz Menéndez Benito. Benign and malignant tumors of the lung: Classification. Diagnosis. Treatment. Rev. Cubana Cir. [Internet]. 2019 Dec [cited 2023 Apr 06]; 45(3-4) Available from:

20. https://instituciones.sld.cu/fcmdoct/files/2019/02/Clasificacion-diagnostico-de-tumoresbenignos-y-malignos-del-pulmon.pdf

21. PAHO/WHO. Lung Cancer in the Americas.2022. [cited 2023 Apr 06]; Available from: https://www.paho.org/es/temas/cancer

22. Demographic Yearbook of Cuba. January-December 2022. . [cited 2023 Apr 06]; Available from: https://www.onei.gob.cu/anuario-demografico-de-cuba-enero-diciembre-2022

23. González R, Barra S, Riquelme A. Lung cancer characterization, staging and survival in the Chilean public health system Hospital.Rev.med.Chile vol.150.1 [Internet]. 2022. [cited 2023 Dec] Available from: https://www.scielo.cl/scielo.php?script=sci_arttext&pid=S0034-98872022000100007

24. Cabo García A, Del Campo Mulet E, Rubio González T, Nápoles Smith N, Columbie Reguifero JC. Clinical and epidemiological aspects in patients with lung cancer in a pulmonology service. MEDISAN [Internet]. 2018 Apr [cited 2024 Apr 19]; 22(4): 394-405. Available from: http://scielo.sld.cu/scielo.php?script=sci_arttext&pid=S1029-30192018000400009&lng=es.

25. Machandi Thomas O, Cristiá Lara S. Demographic characterization of Guantánamo province (2013-2017). Rev Noved Poblac [Internet]. 2020 [Cited 2024 Apr 19]; 16(31): 127-137. Available at: http:

26. Galano AS, Paumier ZT, Antúnez, MBP. Cancer mortality in adult population of Baracoa. Rev Informa Cient [Internet]. 2011 [Cited 2024 Apr 19]; 69(1):1-11 Available from: https:

27. Rousseaux Modesi A, Blanco García L, Reyes Pacheco A, Sánchez Reyes R, Baglán Acosta B. Mortality by malignant tumors in the Policlínico Universitario" 4 de Abril" of Guantánamo municipality. Rev Info Cient [Internet]. 2013 [Cited 2024 Apr 19]; *77*(1):1-13 Available from: https:

28. Etienne CF. Tobacco control in the Americas: what's missing, what's next? Rev Panam Public Health. [Internet]. 2022 [Cited 2024 Apr 19]; 46:e160. https://doi.org/10.26633/RPSP.2022.160Disponible at: https://www.scielosp.org/article/rpsp/2022.v46/e160/es/

29. Cahuana Pinto, R. Systematic review and meta-analysis on the risk of lung cancer in workers in the civil construction industry. [Internet]. Corporación Barranquilla Colombia Universidad de la Costa; 2020 [cited: 2024, April] Available from: https:

30. Jiménez Massa AE. Lung cancer and cytokines: clinical and genetic variants. [Thesis in option to the title of Doctor] [Internet]. Salamanca Spain, University of Salamanca; 2011 [Cited 2024 Apr 19] Available from: https:

31. Gómez-Tejeda J, Tamayo-Velazquez O, Iparraguirre-Tamayo A, Dieguez-Guach R. Behavior of risk factors for lung neoplasia. Universidad Médica Pinareña [journal on the Internet]. 2020 [cited 19 Apr 2024]; 16 (3) Available from: https:

32. Santos Concepción ID. Main risk factors in patients with lung cancer in the Territorial Oncology Center of Holguin. 2020-2022 [Thesis in option to the title of First Degree Specialist in Medical Oncology] [Internet]. Holguín Cuba Universidad Ciencias Médicas de Holguín; 2022 [Cited 2024 Apr 19] Available from: https://tesis.hlg.sld.cu/index.php?P=FullRecord&ID=3214

33. Giraldo-Osorio A, Ruano-Ravina A, Rey-Brandariz J, Arias-Ortiz N, Candal-Pedreira C, Pérez-Ríos M. Trends in lung cancer mortality in Colombia, 1985-2018. Rev Panam Salud Publica. [Internet]. 2022 [Cited 2024 Apr 19];46:e127 Available from: https:

34. Zambrano Cedeño AA, Perero Cobeña YS, Castro Jalca J. Risk factors for Lung Cancer: Global impact on the population. Rev Hig de la Salud [Internet]. 2022 [Cited 2024 Apr 19]; 7(2):13-31 Available from: https:

35. Quispe Rodriguez GH. Lung cancer: clinical epidemiological and sociodemographic characteristics in the hospital Antonio Lorena del Cusco, 2015-2021 [Thesis in option to the degree of Medical Surgeon] [Internet]. Cusco Peru, Universidad Nacional San Antonio Abad del Cusco; 2022 [Cited 2024 Apr 19] Available from: http:

36. Pérez García S, Pérez García S, Ramos Cordero AE, Junco Labrador L, Hernández Gómez E Characterization of patients with lung cancer in Policlínico Universitario "Fermín Valdés Domínguez "de Viñales. Rev Corr Cient Med [Internet]. 2022 ci 2024 Apr 19]; *26*(2):1-11 Available in: https:

37. Motta Guerrero R, Huerta-Collado Y, Failoc-Rojas VE, Cabezas Orellana DC, Leon Garrido-Lecca A, Calle-Villavicencio A, Torres-Mera A, Valladares-Garrido MJ, Aliaga Macha C, Carracedo C. Epidemiological and molecular profile of patients with lung cancer in a referral cancer center in Lima, Peru . Rev. Cuerpo Med. HNAAA [Internet]. November 5, 2023 [cited April 19, 2024];16(3). Available from: https:

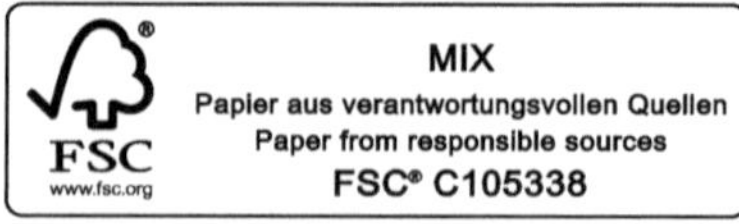

Printed by Books on Demand GmbH, Norderstedt / Germany